Easy Plant-Ba Recipes For Be...

A Beginners Plant-Based Diet Cookbook with Practical Recipes to Get Started in the Kitchen, a Better Way to Cook Great Food and Losing Weight

Virginia Larson

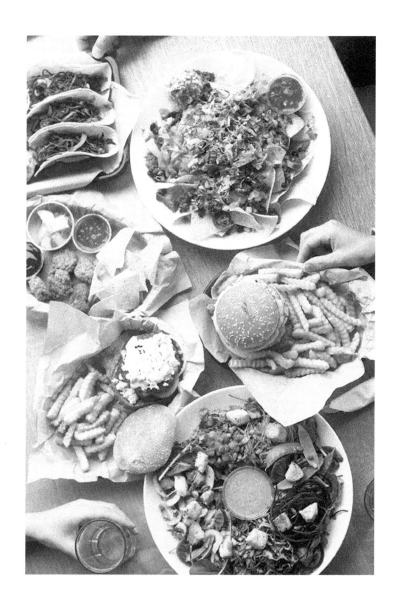

Table of Contents

The information in the following pages is broadly considered a truthful and accurate account of facts and as such, any inattention, use, or misuse of the information in question by the reader will render any resulting actions solely under their purview. There are no scenarios in which the publisher or the original author of this work can be in any fashion deemed liable for any hardship or damages that may befall them after undertaking information described herein.

Additionally, the information in the following pages is intended only for informational purposes and should thus be thought of as universal. As befitting its nature, it is presented without assurance regarding its prolonged validity or interim quality. Trademarks that are mentioned are done without written consent and can in no way be considered an endorsement from the trademark holder.

Introduction

A plant-based diet is a diet based primarily on whole plant foods. It is identical to the regular diet we're used to already, except that it leaves out foods that are not exclusively from plants. Hence, a plant-based diet does away with all types of animal-sourced foods, hydrogenated oils, refined sugars, and processed foods. A whole food plant-based diet comprises not just fruits and vegetables; it also consists of unprocessed or barely-processed oils with healthy monounsaturated fats (like extra-virgin olive oil), whole grains, legumes (essentially lentils and beans), seeds and nuts, as well as herbs and spices.

What makes a plant-based meal (or any meal) fun is the manner with which you make them; the seasoning process; and the combination process that contributes to a fantastic flavor and makes every meal unique and enjoyable. There are lots of delicious recipes (all plant-centered), which will prove helpful in when you intend making mouthwatering, healthy plant-based dishes for personal or household consumption. Provided you're eating these plant-based foods regularly, you'll have very problems with fat or diseases that result from bad dietary habits, and there would be no need for excessive calorie tracking.

Plant-based diet recipes are versatile; they range from colorful Salads to Lentil Stews, and Bean Burritos. The recipes also draw influences from around the globe, with Mexican, Chinese, European, Indian cuisines all part of the vast array of plant-based recipes available to choose from. Why You Ought to Reduce Your Intake of Processed and Animal-Based Foods. You have likely heard over and over that processed food has adverse effects on your health. You might have also been told repeatedly to stay away from foods with lots of preservatives; nevertheless, nobody ever offered any genuine or concrete facts about why you ought to avoid these foods and why they are unsafe. Consequently, let us properly dissect it to help you properly comprehend why you ought to stay away from these healthy eating offenders. They have massive habit-forming characteristics. Humans have a predisposition towards being addicted to some specific foods; however, the reality is that the fault is not wholly ours. Every one of the unhealthy treats we relish now and then triggers the dopamine release in our brains. This creates a pleasurable effect in our brain, but the excitement is usually short-lived. The discharged dopamine additionally causes an attachment connection gradually, and this is the reason some people consistently go back to eat certain unhealthy foods even when they know it's unhealthy and unnecessary.

You can get rid of this by taking out that inducement completely. They are sugar-laden and plenteous in glucose-fructose syrup. Animal-based and processed foods are laden with refined sugars and glucose-fructose syrup which has almost no beneficial food nutrient. An ever-increasing number of studies are affirming what several people presumed from the start; that genetically modified foods bring about inflammatory bowel disease, which consequently makes it increasingly difficult for the body to assimilate essential nutrients. The disadvantages that result from your body being unable to assimilate essential nutrients from consumed foods rightly cannot be overemphasized. Processed and animal-based food products contain plenteous amounts of refined carbohydrates. Indeed, your body requires carbohydrates to give it the needed energy to run body capacities. In any case, refining carbs dispenses with the fundamental supplements; in the way that refining entire grains disposes of the whole grain part. What remains, in the wake of refining, is what's considered as empty carbs or empty calories. These can negatively affect the metabolic system in your body by sharply increasing your blood sugar and insulin quantities. They contain lots of synthetic ingredients. At the point when your body is taking in non-natural ingredients, it regards them as foreign substances.

Your body treats them as a health threat. Your body isn't accustomed to identifying synthetic compounds like sucralose or these synthesized sugars. Hence, in defense of your health against this foreign "aggressor," your body does what it's capable of to safeguard your health. It sets off an immune reaction to tackle this "enemy" compound, which indirectly weakens your body's general disease alertness, making you susceptible to illnesses. The concentration and energy expended by your body in ensuring your immune system remain safe could instead be devoted somewhere else. They contain constituent elements that set off an excitable reward sensation in your body. A part of processed and animal-based foods contain compounds like glucose-fructose syrup, monosodium glutamate, and specific food dyes that can trigger some addiction. They rouse your body to receive a benefit in return whenever you consume them. Monosodium glutamate, for example, is added to many store-bought baked foods. This additive slowly conditions your palates to relish the taste. It gets mental just by how your brain interrelates with your taste sensors.

This reward-centric arrangement makes you crave it increasingly, which ends up exposing you to the danger of over consuming calories.

For animal protein, usually, the expression "subpar" is used to allude to plant proteins since they generally have lower levels of essential amino acids as against animal-sourced protein. Nevertheless, what the vast majority don't know is that large amounts of essential amino acids can prove detrimental to your health. Let me break it down further for you.

Stuffed Sweet Potatoes

Preparation Time: 30 minutes

Cooking Time: 21 minutes

Serving: 3

Ingredients:

- ½ cup dry black beans
- 3 small or medium sweet potatoes
- 2 tbsp. olive oil
- 1 large red bell pepper, pitted, chopped
- 1 small sweet yellow onion, chopped
- 2 tbsp. garlic, minced or powdered
- 1 8-oz. package tempeh, diced into ¼" cubes
- ½ cup marinara sauce
- ½ cup water
- 1 tbsp. chili powder
- 1 tsp. parsley
- ½ tsp. cayenne
- ¼ tsp Salt
- ¼ tsp pepper

Directions:

1. Preheat the oven to 400°F.

2. Using a fork, stab several holes in the skins of the sweet potatoes.

3. Wrap the sweet potatoes tightly with aluminum foil and place them in the oven until soft and tender, or for approximately 45 minutes.

4. While sweet potatoes are cooking, heat the olive oil in a deep pan over medium-high heat. Add the onions, bell peppers, and garlic; cook until the onions are tender, for about 10 minutes.

5. Add the water, together with the cooked beans, marinara sauce, chili powder, parsley, and cayenne. Bring the mixture to a boil and then lower the heat to medium or low. Allow the mixture to simmer until the liquid has thickened, for about 15 minutes.

6. Add the diced tempeh cubes and heat until warmed, around 1 minute.

7. Blend in salt and pepper to taste.

8. When the potatoes are done baking, get rid of them from the oven. Cut a slit across the top of each one, but do not split the potatoes in half.

9. Top each potato with a scoop of the beans, vegetables, and tempeh mixture. Place the filled potatoes back in the hot oven for about 5 minutes.

10. Serve after cooling for a few minutes, or, store for another day!

Nutrition:

Calories 548, Total Fat 19.7g, Cholesterol 1mg, Sodium 448mg, Total Carbohydrate 76g, Dietary Fiber 12.4g, Total Sugars 15.2g, Protein 25.3g, Vitamin D 0mcg, Calcium 185mg, Iron 5mg, Potassium 1132mg

Roasted Cauliflower

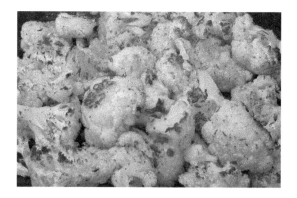

Preparation Time: 5 minutes

Cooking time: 15 minutes

Servings: 2

Ingredients:

- Medium head cauliflower

- 2 tablespoon salted butter, melted

- 1 medium lemon

- 1 teaspoon dried parsley

- 1/2 teaspoon garlic powder

Directions:

1. Having removed the leaves from the cauliflower head, brush it with the melted butter.

2. Grate the rind of the lemon over it and then drizzle some juice. Finally add the parsley and garlic powder on top.

3. Transfer the cauliflower to the basket of the fryer.

4. Cook for fifteen minutes at 350°F, checking regularly to ensure it doesn't overcook. The cauliflower is ready when it is hot and fork tender.

5. Take care when removing it from the fryer, cut up and serve.

Nutrition:

Calories: 270

Fat: 20g

Carbs: 5g

Protein: 3g

Forest Mushroom Loaf

Preparation Time: 5 minutes

Cooking time: 15 minutes

Servings: 2

Ingredients:

- 2 cups mushrooms, chopped

- 1/2 cups vegan cheese, shredded

- 3/4 cup flour

- 2 tablespoon butter, melted

- 2 eggs

Directions:

1. In a food processor, pulse together the mushrooms, cheese, flour, melted butter, and eggs, along with some salt and pepper if desired, until a uniform consistency is achieved.

2. Transfer into a silicone loaf pan, spreading and levelling with a palette knife.

3. Pre-heat the fryer at 375 degree Fahrenheit and put the rack inside.

4. Set the loaf pan on the rack and cook for fifteen minutes.

5. Take care when removing the pan from the fryer and leave it to cool. Then slice and serve.

Nutrition:

Calories: 205

Fat: 5g

Carbs: 8g

Protein: 4g

Green Bean Casserole

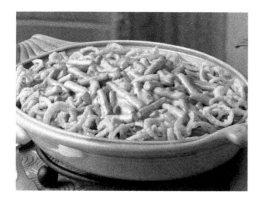

Preparation Time: 5 minutes

Cooking time: 5 minutes

Servings: 2

Ingredients:

- Tablespoon butter, melted

- 1 cup green beans

- 6 oz. vegan cheese, shredded

- 1/4 cup heavy vegan cream

Directions:

1. Pre-heat your fryer at 400 degree Fahrenheit.

2. Take a baking dish small enough to fit inside the fryer and cover the bottom with melted butter.

3. Throw in the green beans, vegan cheese, and any seasoning as desired, then give it a stir.

4. Add the parmesan on top and finally the heavy cream.

5. Cook in the fryer for six minutes. Allow to cool before serving.

Nutrition:

Calories: 190

Fat: 16g

Carbs: 5g

Protein: 7g

Cabbage Steaks

Preparation Time: 5 minutes

Cooking time: 5 minutes

Servings: 2

Ingredients:

- Small head cabbage

- 1 teaspoon butter, butter

- 1 teaspoon paprika

- 1 teaspoon olive oil

Directions:

1. Halve the cabbage.

2. In a bowl, mix the melted butter, paprika, and olive oil.

3. Massage into the cabbage slices, making sure to coat it well.

4. Season as desired with salt and pepper or any other seasonings of you're choosing.

5. Pre-heat the fryer at 400 degree Fahrenheit and set the rack inside.

6. Put the cabbage in the fryer and cook for three minutes. Flip it and cook on the other side for another two minutes. Enjoy!

Nutrition:

Calories: 170

Fat: 10g

Carbs: 9g

Protein: 7g

Dinner Recipes

Instant Savory Gigante Beans

Preparation Time: 10-30 minutes

Cooking Time: 55 minutes

Servings: 6

Ingredients:

- 1 lb Gigante Beans soaked overnight

- 1/2 cup olive oil

- 1 onion sliced

- 2 cloves garlic crushed or minced

- 1 red bell pepper (cut into 1/2-inch pieces)

- 2 carrots, sliced

- 1/2 teaspoon salt and ground black pepper

- 2 tomatoes peeled, grated

- 1 Tablespoon celery (chopped)

- 1 Tablespoon tomato paste (or ketchup)

- 3/4 teaspoon sweet paprika

- 1 teaspoon oregano

- 1 cup vegetable broth

Directions:

1. Soak Gigante beans overnight.

2. Press SAUTÉ button on your Instant Pot and heat the oil.

3. Sauté onion, garlic, sweet pepper, carrots with a pinch of salt for 3 - 4 minutes; stir occasionally.

4. Add rinsed Gigante beans into your Instant Pot along with all remaining **Ingredients:** and stir well.

5. Lock lid into place and set on the MANUAL setting for 25 minutes.

6. When the beep sounds, quick release the pressure by pressing Cancel, and twisting the steam handle to the Venting position.

7. Taste and adjust seasonings to taste.

8. Serve warm or cold.

Keep refrigerated.

Nutrition:

Calories 502.45,

Total Fat 19.63g,

Saturated Fat 2.86g

Instant Turmeric Risotto

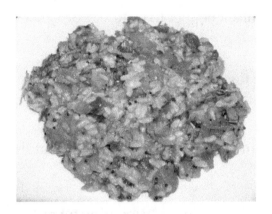

Preparation Time: 10-30 minutes

Cooking Time: 40 minutes

Servings: 4

Ingredients:

- 4 Tablespoon olive oil

- 1 cup onion

- 1 teaspoon minced garlic

- 2 cups long-grain rice

- 3 cups vegetable broth

- 1/2 teaspoon paprika (smoked)

- 1/2 teaspoon turmeric

- 1/2 teaspoon nutmeg

- 2 Tablespoon fresh basil leaves chopped

- Salt and ground black pepper to taste

Directions:

1. Press the SAUTÉ button on your Instant Pot and heat oil.

2. Sauté the onion and garlic with a pinch of salt until softened.

3. Add the rice and all remaining **Ingredients:** and stir well.

4. Lock lid into place and set on and select the "RICE" button for 10 minutes.

5. Press "Cancel" when the timer beeps and carefully flip the Quick Release valve to let the pressure out.

6. Taste and adjust seasonings to taste.

7. Serve.

Nutrition:

Calories 559.81,

Calories from Fat 162.48,

Total Fat 18.57g,

Saturated Fat 2.4g

Nettle Soup with Rice

Preparation Time: 10-30 minutes
Cooking Time: 40 minutes
Servings: 5
Ingredients:

- 3 Tablespoon of olive oil

- 2 onions finely chopped

- 2 cloves garlic finely chopped

- Salt and freshly ground black pepper

- 4 medium potatoes cut into cubes

- 1 cup of rice

- 1 Tablespoon arrowroot

- 2 cups vegetable broth

- 2 cups of water

- 1 bunch of young nettle leaves packed

- 1/2 cup fresh parsley finely chopped

- 1 teaspoon cumin

Directions:
1. Heat olive oil in a large pot.

2. Sauté onion and garlic with a pinch of salt until softened.

3. Add potato, rice, and arrowroot; sauté for 2 to 3 minutes.

4. Pour broth and water, stir well, cover and cook over medium heat for about 20 minutes.

5. Cook over medium heat for about 20 minutes.

6. Add young nettle leaves, parsley, and cumin; stir and cook for 5 to 7 minutes.

7. Transfer the soup in a blender and blend until combined well.

8. Taste and adjust salt and pepper.

9. Serve hot.

Nutrition:

Calories 421.76

Calories from Fat 88.32

Total Fat 9.8g

Saturated Fat 1.54g

Okra with Grated Tomatoes (Slow Cooker)

Preparation Time: 10-30 minutes
Cooking Time: 3 hours and 10 minutes
Servings: 4
Ingredients:

- 2 lbs fresh okra cleaned

- 2 onions finely chopped

- 2 cloves garlic finely sliced

- 2 carrots sliced

- 2 ripe tomatoes grated

- 1 cup of water

- 4 Tablespoon olive oil

- Salt and ground black pepper

- 1 Tablespoon fresh parsley finely chopped

Directions:

1. Add okra in your Crock-Pot: sprinkle with a pinch of salt and pepper.

2. Add in chopped onion, garlic, carrots, and grated tomatoes; stir well.

3. Pour water and oil, season with the salt, pepper, and give a good stir.

4. Cover and cook on LOW for 2-3 hours or until tender.

5. Open the lid and add fresh parsley; stir.

6. Taste and adjust salt and pepper.

7. Serve hot.

Nutrition:

Calories 223.47

Calories from Fat 123.5

Total Fat 14g

Saturated Fat 1.96g

Oven-baked Smoked Lentil 'Burgers'

Preparation Time: 10-30 minutes
Cooking Time: 1 hour and 20 minutes
Servings: 6
Ingredients:

- 1 1/2 cups dried lentils

- 3 cups of water

- Salt and ground black pepper to taste

- 2 Tablespoon olive oil

- 1 onion finely diced

- 2 cloves minced garlic

- 1 cup button mushrooms sliced

- 2 Tablespoon tomato paste

- 1/2 teaspoon fresh basil finely chopped

- 1 cup chopped almonds

- 3 teaspoon balsamic vinegar

- 3 Tablespoon coconut aminos

- 1 teaspoon liquid smoke

- 3/4 cup silken tofu soft

- 3/4 cup corn starch

Directions:

1. Cook lentils in salted water until tender or for about 30-35 minutes; rinse, drain, and set aside.

2. Heat oil in a frying skillet and sauté onion, garlic and mushrooms for 4 to 5 minutes; stir occasionally.

3. Stir in the tomato paste, salt, basil, salt, and black pepper; cook for 2 to 3 minutes.

4. Stir in almonds, vinegar, coconut aminos, liquid smoke, and lentils.

5. Remove from heat and stir in blended tofu and corn starch.

6. Keep stirring until all **Ingredients:** combined well.

7. Form mixture into patties and refrigerate for an hour.

8. Preheat oven to 350 F.

9. Line a baking dish with parchment paper and arrange patties on the pan.

10. Bake for 20 to 25 minutes.

11. Serve hot with buns, green salad, tomato sauce...etc.

Nutrition:

Calories 439.12

Calories from Fat 148.97

Total Fat 17.48g

Saturated Fat 1.71g

Powerful Spinach and Mustard Leaves Puree

Preparation Time: 10-30 minutes

Cooking Time: 50 minutes

Servings: 4

Ingredients:

- 2 Tablespoon almond butter

- 1 onion finely diced

- 2 Tablespoon minced garlic

- 1 teaspoon salt and black pepper (or to taste)

- 1 lb mustard leaves, cleaned rinsed

- 1 lb frozen spinach thawed

- 1 teaspoon coriander

- 1 teaspoon ground cumin

- 1/2 cup almond milk

Directions:

1. Press the SAUTÉ button on your Instant Pot and heat the almond butter.

2. Sauté onion, garlic, and a pinch of salt for 2-3 minutes; stir occasionally.

3. Add spinach and the mustard greens and stir for a minute or two.

4. Season with the salt and pepper, coriander, and cumin; give a good stir.

5. Lock lid into place and set on the MANUAL setting for 15 minutes.

6. Use Quick Release - turn the valve from sealing to venting to release the pressure.

7. Transfer mixture to a blender, add almond milk and blend until smooth.

8. Taste and adjust seasonings.

9. Serve.

Nutrition:

Calories 180.53

Calories from Fat 82.69

Total Fat 10g

Saturated Fat 0.65g

Quinoa and Rice Stuffed Peppers (oven-baked)

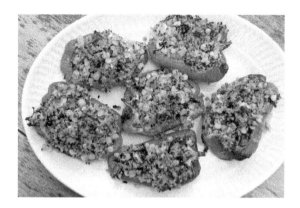

Preparation Time: 10-30 minutes

Cooking Time: 35 minutes

Servings: 8

Ingredients:

- 3/4 cup long-grain rice

- 8 bell peppers (any color)

- 2 Tablespoon olive oil

- 1 onion finely diced

- 2 cloves chopped garlic

- 1 can (11 oz) crushed tomatoes

- 1 teaspoon cumin

- 1 teaspoon coriander

- 4 Tablespoon ground walnuts

- 2 cups cooked quinoa

- 4 Tablespoon chopped parsley

- Salt and ground black pepper to taste

Directions:

1. Preheat oven to 400 F/200 C.

2. Boil rice and drain in a colander.

3. Cut the top stem section of the pepper off, remove the remaining pith and seeds, rinse peppers.

4. Heat oil in a large frying skillet, and sauté onion and garlic until soft.

5. Add tomatoes, cumin, ground almonds, salt, pepper, and coriander; stir well and simmer for 2 minutes stirring constantly.

6. Remove from the heat and add the rice, quinoa, and parsley; stir well.

7. Taste and adjust salt and pepper.

8. Fill the peppers with a mixture, and place peppers cut side-up in a baking dish; drizzle with little oil.

9. Bake for 15 minutes.

10. Serve warm.

Nutrition:

Calories 335.69

Calories from Fat 83.63

Total Fat 9.58g

Saturated Fat 1.2g

Quinoa and Lentils with Crushed Tomato

Preparation Time: 10-30 minutes
Cooking Time: 35 minutes
Servings: 4
Ingredients:

- 4 Tablespoon olive oil

- 1 medium onion, diced

- 2 garlic clove, minced

- Salt and ground black pepper to taste

- 1 can (15 oz) tomatoes crushed

- 1 cup vegetable broth

- 1/2 cup quinoa, washed and drained

- 1 cup cooked lentils

- 1 teaspoon chili powder

- 1 teaspoon cumin

Directions:

1. Heat oil in a pot and sauté the onion and garlic with the pinch of salt until soft.

2. Pour reserved tomatoes and vegetable broth, bring to boil, and stir well.

3. Stir in the quinoa, cover and cook for 15 minutes; stir occasionally.

4. Add in lentils, chili powder, and cumin; cook for further 5 minutes.

5. Taste and adjust seasonings.

6. Serve immediately.

7. Keep refrigerated in a covered container for 4 - 5 days.

Nutrition:

Calories: 397.45

Calories from Fat: 138.18

Total Fat: 15.61g

Saturated Fat: 2.14g

Silk Tofu Penne with Spinach

Preparation Time: 10-30 minutes

Cooking Time: 25 minutes

Servings: 4

Ingredients:

- 1 lb penne, uncooked

- 12 oz of frozen spinach, thawed

- 1 cup silken tofu mashed

- 1/2 cup soy milk (unsweetened)

- 1/2 cup vegetable broth

- 1 Tablespoon white wine vinegar

- 1/2 teaspoon Italian seasoning

- Salt and ground pepper to taste

Directions:

1. Cook penne pasta; rinse and drain in a colander.

2. Drain spinach well.

3. Place spinach with all remaining **Ingredients:** in a blender and beat until smooth.

4. Pour the spinach mixture over pasta.

5. Taste and adjust the salt and pepper.

6. Store pasta in an airtight container in the refrigerator for 3 to 5 days.

Nutrition:

Calories: 492.8

Calories from Fat: 27.06

Total Fat: 3.07g

Saturated Fat: 0.38g

Super Radish Avocado Salad

Preparation time: 10 minutes

Cooking time: 25 minutes

Servings: 2 Salads.

Ingredients:

- 6 shredded carrots

- 6 ounces diced radishes

- 1 diced avocado

- 1/3 cup ponzu

Directions:

1. Bring all the above **Ingredients:** together in a serving bowl and toss. Enjoy!

Nutrition:

Calories: 211

Carbs: 9g

Fat: 7g

Protein: 12g

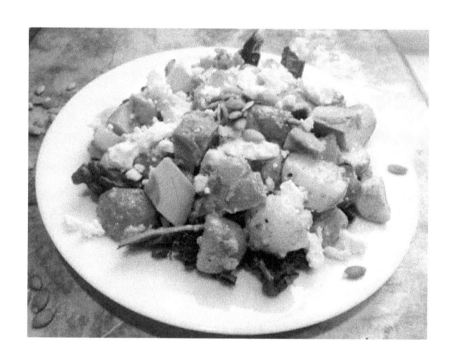

Soya Minced Stuffed Eggplants

Preparation Time: 10-30 minutes
Cooking Time: 1 hour, **Servings:** 4
Ingredients:

- 2 eggplants

- 1/3 cup sesame oil

- 1 onion finely chopped

- 2 garlic cloves minced

- 1 lb soya mince* see note

- Salt and ground black pepper

- 1/3 cup almond milk

- 2 Tablespoon fresh parsley, chopped

- 1/3 cup fresh basil chopped

- 1 teaspoon fennel powder

- 1 cup of water

- 4 Tablespoon tomato paste (fresh or canned)

Directions:

1. Rinse and slice the eggplant in half lengthwise.

2. Submerge sliced eggplant into a container with salted water.

3. Soak soya mince in water for 10 to 15 minutes.

4. Preheat oven to 400 F.

5. Rinse eggplant and dry with a clean towel.

6. Heat oil in large frying skillet, and sauté onion and garlic with a pinch of salt until softened.

7. Add drained soya mince, and cook over medium heat until cooked through.

8. Add all remaining **Ingredients:** (except water and tomato paste) and cook for a further 5 minutes; remove from heat.

9. Scoop out the seed part of each eggplant.

10. Spoon in the filling and arrange stuffed eggplants onto the large baking dish.

11. Dissolve tomato paste into the water and pour evenly over eggplants.

12. Bake for 20 to 25 minutes.

13. Serve warm.

Nutrition:

Calories: 287.32

Calories from Fat: 141.77

Total Fat: 16.42g

Saturated Fat: 2.02g

Black Bean Burgers

Preparation Time: 10 minutes

Cooking Time: 15 minutes

Servings: 6

Ingredients:

- 1 Onion, diced
- ½ cup Corn Nibs
- 2 Cloves Garlic, minced
- ½ teaspoon Oregano, dried
- ½ cup Flour
- 1 Jalapeno Pepper, small
- 2 cups Black Beans, mashed & canned
- ¼ cup Breadcrumbs (Vegan)
- 2 teaspoons Parsley, minced
- ¼ teaspoon cumin
- 1 tablespoon Olive Oil
- 2 teaspoons Chili Powder
- ½ Red Pepper, diced
- Sea Salt to taste

Directions:

1. Set your flour on a plate, and then get out your garlic, onion, peppers and oregano, throwing it in a pan. Cook over medium-high heat, and

then cook until the onions are translucent. Place the peppers in, and sauté until tender.

2. Cook for two minutes, and then set it to the side.

3. Use a potato masher to mash your black beans, then stir in the vegetables, cumin, breadcrumbs, parsley, salt, and chili powder, and then divide it into six patties.

4. Coat each side, and then cook until it is fried on each side.

Nutrition:

Calories: 357 kcal

Protein: 17.93 g

Fat: 5.14 g

Carbohydrates: 61.64 g

Dijon Maple Burgers

Preparation Time: 20 minutes

Cooking Time: 30 minutes

Servings: 12

Ingredients:

- 1 Red Bell Pepper
- 19 ounces Can Chickpeas, rinsed & drained
- 1 cup Almonds, ground
- 2 teaspoons Dijon Mustard
- 1 teaspoon Oregano
- ½ teaspoon Sage
- 1 cup Spinach, fresh
- 1 – ½ cups Rolled Oats
- 1 Clove Garlic, pressed
- ½ Lemon, juiced
- 2 teaspoons Maple Syrup, pure

Directions:

1. Get out a baking sheet. Line it with parchment paper.
2. Cut your red pepper in half and then take the seeds out. Place it on your baking sheet, and roast in the oven while you prepare your other ingredients.
3. Process your chickpeas, almonds, mustard, and maple syrup together in a food processor.

4. Add in your lemon juice, oregano, sage, garlic, and spinach, processing again. Make sure it's combined, but don't puree it.

5. Once your red bell pepper is softened, which should roughly take ten minutes, add this to the processor as well. Add in your oats, mixing well.

6. Form twelve patties, cooking in the oven for a half-hour. They should be browned.

Nutrition:

Calories: 96 kcal

Protein: 5.28 g

Fat: 2.42 g

Carbohydrates: 16.82 g

Hearty Black Lentil Curry

Preparation Time: 30 minutes

Cooking Time: 6 hours and 15 minutes

Servings: 4

Ingredients:

1 cup of black lentils, rinsed and soaked overnight

14 ounce of chopped tomatoes

2 large white onions, peeled and sliced

1 1/2 teaspoon of minced garlic

1 teaspoon of grated ginger

1 red chili

1 teaspoon of salt

1/4 teaspoon of red chili powder

1 teaspoon of paprika

1 teaspoon of ground turmeric

2 teaspoons of ground cumin

2 teaspoons of ground coriander

1/2 cup of chopped coriander

4-ounce of vegetarian butter

4 fluid of ounce water

2 fluid of ounce vegetarian double cream

Directions:

Place a large pan over moderate heat, add butter and
let heat until melt.

Add the onion and garlic and ginger and cook for 10 to 15 minutes or until onions are caramelized.

Then stir in salt, red chili powder, paprika, turmeric, cumin, ground coriander, and water.

Transfer this mixture to a 6-quarts slow cooker and add tomatoes and red chili.

Drain lentils, add to slow cooker, and stir until just mix.

Plugin slow cooker; adjust cooking time to 6 hours and let cook on low heat setting.

When the lentils are done, stir in cream and adjust the seasoning.

Serve with boiled rice or whole wheat bread.

Nutrition:

Calories: 299 kcal

Protein: 5.59 g

Fat: 27.92 g

Carbohydrates: 9.83 g

Smoky Red Beans and Rice

Preparation Time: 15 minutes

Cooking Time: 6 minutes

Servings: 6

Ingredients:

30 ounce of cooked red beans

1 cup of brown rice, uncooked

1 cup of chopped green pepper

1 cup of chopped celery

1 cup of chopped white onion

1 1/2 teaspoon of minced garlic

1/2 teaspoon of salt

1/4 teaspoon of cayenne pepper

1 teaspoon of smoked paprika

2 teaspoons of dried thyme

1 bay leaf

2 1/3 cups of vegetable broth

Directions:

Using a 6-quarts slow cooker, place all the ingredients except for the rice, salt, and cayenne pepper.

Stir until it mixes properly and then cover the top.

Plug in the slow cooker, adjust the cooking time to 4 hours, and steam on a low heat setting.

Then pour in and stir the rice, salt, cayenne pepper and
continue cooking for an additional 2 hours at a high
heat setting.

Serve straight away.

Nutrition:

Calories: 791 kcal

Protein: 3.25 g

Fat: 86.45 g

Carbohydrates: 9.67 g

Spicy Black-Eyed Peas

Preparation Time: 12 minutes
Cooking Time: 8 hours and 8 minutes
Servings: 8
Ingredients:

32-ounce black-eyed peas, uncooked

1 cup of chopped orange bell pepper

1 cup of chopped celery

8-ounce of chipotle peppers, chopped

1 cup of chopped carrot

1 cup of chopped white onion

1 teaspoon of minced garlic

3/4 teaspoon of salt

1/2 teaspoon of ground black pepper

2 teaspoons of liquid smoke flavoring

2 teaspoons of ground cumin

1 tablespoon of adobo sauce

2 tablespoons of olive oil

1 tablespoon of apple cider vinegar

4 cups of vegetable broth

Directions:

Place a medium-sized non-stick skillet pan over an
average temperature of heat; add the bell peppers,
carrot, onion, garlic, oil, and vinegar.

Stir until it mixes properly and let it cook for 5 to 8 minutes or until it gets translucent.

Transfer this mixture to a 6-quarts slow cooker and add the peas, chipotle pepper, adobo sauce, and the vegetable broth.

Stir until mixed properly and cover the top.

Plug in the slow cooker, adjust the cooking time to 8 hours, and let it cook on the low heat setting or until peas are soft.

Serve right away.

Nutrition:

Calories: 1071 kcal

Protein: 5.3 g

Fat: 113.65 g

Carbohydrates: 18.51 g

Creamy Artichoke Soup

Preparation Time: 5 minutes

Cooking Time: 40 minutes

Servings: 4

Ingredients:

>1 can artichoke hearts, drained
>
>3 cups vegetable broth
>
>2 tbsp. lemon juice
>
>1 small onion, finely cut
>
>2 cloves garlic, crushed
>
>3 tbsp. olive oil
>
>2 tbsp. flour
>
>½ cup vegan cream

Directions:

>Gently sauté the onion and garlic in some olive oil. Add the flour, whisking constantly, and then add the hot vegetable broth slowly, while still whisking. Cook for about 5 minutes.
>
>Blend the artichoke, lemon juice, salt, and pepper until smooth. Add the puree to the broth mix, stir well, and then stir in the cream. Cook until heated through. Garnish with a swirl of vegan cream or a sliver of artichoke.

Nutrition:

Calories: 1622 kcal

Protein: 4.45 g

Fat: 181.08 g

Carbohydrates: 10.99 g

Tomato Artichoke Soup

Preparation Time: 5 minutes

Cooking Time: 35 minutes

Servings: 4

Ingredients:

> 1 can artichoke hearts, drained
>
> 1 can diced tomatoes, undrained
>
> 3 cups vegetable broth
>
> 1 small onion, chopped
>
> 2 cloves garlic, crushed
>
> 1 tbsp. pesto
>
> Black pepper, to taste

Directions:

> Combine all ingredients in the slow cooker.
>
> Cover and cook on low for 8-10 hours or on high for 4-5 hours.
>
> Blend the soup in batches then put it back to the slow cooker. Season with pepper and salt, then serve.

Nutrition:

Calories: 1487 kcal

Protein: 3.98 g

Fat: 167.42 g

Carbohydrates: 8.2 g

Beauty School Ginger Cucumbers

Preparation Time: 10 minutes

Cooking Time: 45 minutes

Servings: 14

Ingredients:

> 1 sliced cucumber
>
> 3 tsp. rice wine vinegar
>
> 1 ½ tbsp. sugar
>
> 1 tsp. minced ginger

Directions:

> Place all together the ingredients in a mixing bowl, and toss the ingredients well. Enjoy!

Nutrition:

Calories: 10 kcal

Protein: 0.46 g

Fat: 0.43 g

Carbohydrates: 0.89 g

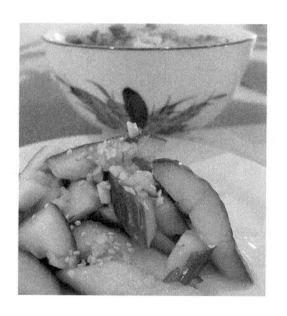

Exotic Butternut Squash and Chickpea Curry

Preparation Time: 20 minutes

Cooking Time: 6 hours

Servings: 8

Ingredients:

- 1 1/2 cups of shelled peas
- 1 1/2 cups of chickpeas, uncooked and rinsed
- 2 1/2 cups of diced butternut squash
- 12 ounce of chopped spinach
- 2 large tomatoes, diced
- 1 small white onion, peeled and chopped
- 1 teaspoon of minced garlic
- 1 teaspoon of salt
- 3 tablespoons of curry powder
- 14-ounce of coconut milk
- 3 cups of vegetable broth
- 1/4 cup of chopped cilantro

Directions:

Using a 6-quarts slow cooker, place all the ingredients into it except for the spinach and peas.

Cover the top, plug in the slow cooker; adjust the cooking time to 6 hours, and cook on the high heat setting or until the chickpeas get tender.

30 minutes to ending your cooking, add the peas and
spinach to the slow cooker and cook for the
remaining 30 minutes.

Stir to check the sauce; if the sauce is runny, stir in a
mixture of a 1 tbsp. Cornstarch mixed with 2 tbsp.
Water.

Serve with boiled rice.

Nutrition:

Calories: 774 kcal

Protein: 3.71 g

Fat: 83.25 g

Carbohydrates: 12.64 g

Sage Walnuts and Radishes

Preparation Time: 10 minutes

Cooking Time: 10 minutes

Servings: 6

Ingredients:

2 tablespoons olive oil

5 celery ribs, chopped

3 spring onions, chopped

½ pound radishes, halved

juice of 1 lime

Zest of 1 lime, grated

8 ounces walnuts, chopped

A pinch of black pepper

3 tablespoons sage, chopped

Directions:

1. Heat up a pan with the oil over medium heat, add celery and spring onion, stir and cook for 5 minutes.

Add the rest of the ingredients, toss, cook for another 5 minutes, divide into bowls and serve.

Nutrition:

Calories 200,Fat 7,Fiber 5,Carbs 9.3, Protein 4

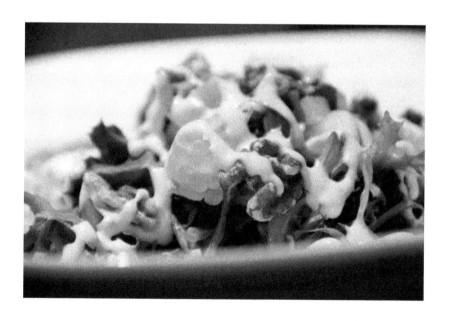

Garlic Zucchini and Cauliflower

Preparation Time: 10 minutes

Cooking Time: 20 minutes

Servings: 4

Ingredients:

- 4 zucchinis, cut into medium fries
- 1 cup cauliflower florets
- 1 tablespoon capers, drained
- Juice of ½ lemon
- A pinch of salt and black pepper
- ½ teaspoon chili powder
- 1 tablespoon olive oil
- ¼ teaspoon garlic powder

Directions:

1. Spread the zucchini fries on a lined baking sheet, add the rest of the ingredients, toss, introduce in the oven, bake at 400 degrees F for 20 minutes, divide between plates and serve.

Nutrition:

Calories 185,Fat 3,Fiber 2,Carbs 6.5, Protein 8

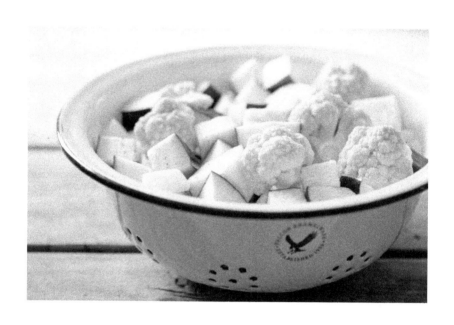

Mustard Beets

Preparation Time: 10 minutes

Cooking Time: 0 minutes

Servings: 4

Ingredients:

> 1 tablespoon Dijon mustard
>
> 1 and ½ tablespoon olive oil
>
> 8 ounces beets, cooked and sliced
>
> 1 teaspoon garam masala
>
> 1 teaspoon coriander, ground
>
> 1 teaspoon basil, dried
>
> A pinch of black pepper

Directions:

In a bowl, mix the beets with the oil, mustard and the other ingredients, toss and serve.

Nutrition:

Calories 170

Fat 5

Fiber 7

Carbs 8

Proteins 5.5

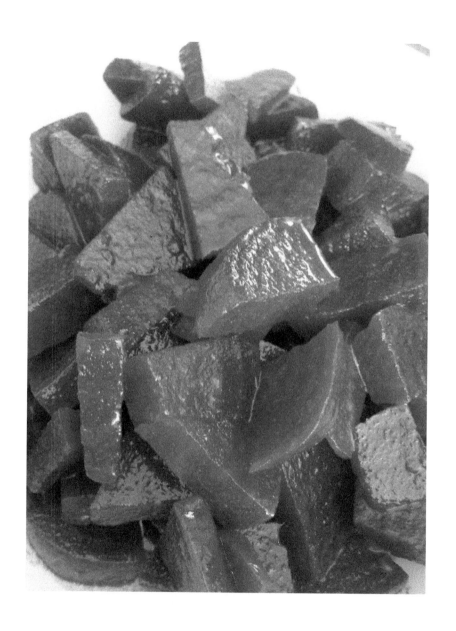

Parsley Green Beans

Preparation Time: 10 minutes

Cooking Time: 20 minutes

Servings: 6

Ingredients:

> 3 tablespoons olive oil
>
> 3 pounds green beans, halved
>
> A pinch of salt and black pepper
>
> 2 tablespoons balsamic vinegar
>
> 2 yellow onions, chopped
>
> 2 and ½ tablespoons parsley, chopped

Directions:

Heat up a pan with the oil over medium heat, add the green beans and the other ingredients, toss, cook for 20 minutes, divide between plates and serve.

Nutrition:

Calories 130

Fat 1

Fiber 2

Carbs 7.4

Protein 6

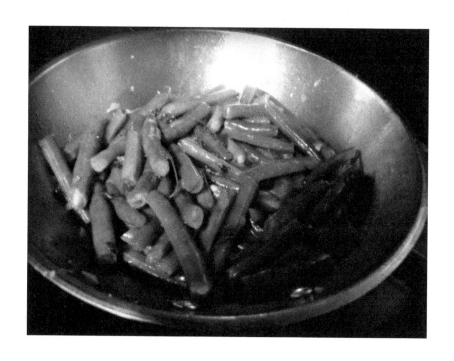

Squash and Tomatoes

Preparation Time: 15 minutes

Cooking Time: 12 minutes

Servings: 2

Ingredients:

> 8 oz yellow squash, peeled and roughly cubed
>
> 1 cup cherry tomatoes, halved
>
> 3 tablespoons tomato sauce
>
> 1 teaspoon sweet paprika
>
> 1 teaspoon coriander, ground
>
> 1 teaspoon oregano, dried
>
> 1 teaspoon olive oil
>
> 1 teaspoon white pepper

Directions:

> Heat up a pan with the oil over medium heat, add the squash, tomatoes and the other ingredients, toss, cook for 12 minutes, divide between plates and serve.

Nutrition:

Calories 41

Fat 2.6

Fiber 1.5

Carbs 4.5 - Protein 1.5

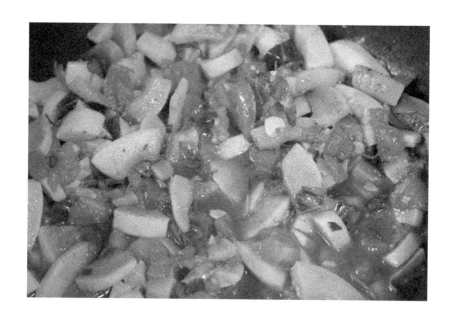

Bok Choy Salad

Preparation Time: 10 minutes

Cooking Time: 10 minutes

Servings: 5

Ingredients:

- 10 oz bok choy, chopped
- 1 cup cherry tomatoes, halved
- 1 tablespoon black olives, pitted and sliced
- 1 mango, peeled and cubed
- Juice of ½ orange
- 1 teaspoon curry powder
- 1 teaspoon sesame oil
- 1 tablespoon lemon juice

Directions:

Heat up a pan with the oil over medium-high heat, add the bok choy, tomatoes and the other ingredients, toss and cook for 10 minutes.

Divide into bowls and serve cold.

Nutrition:

Calories 142,Fat 6.8,Fiber 0.7,Carbs 1.8

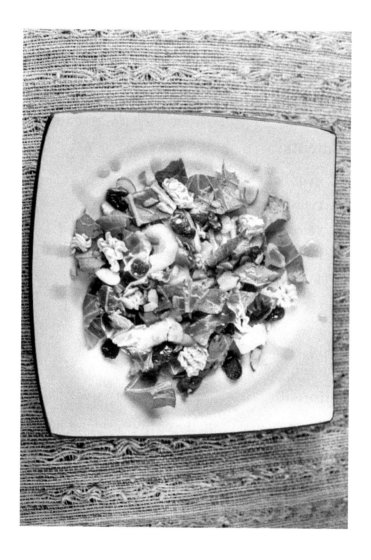

Balsamic Arugula and Beets

Preparation Time: 10 minutes

Cooking Time: 0 minutes

Servings: 4

Ingredients:

> 2 cups baby arugula
>
> 1 tablespoon balsamic vinegar
>
> 1 teaspoon olive oil
>
> 2 red beets, baked, peeled and cubed
>
> 1 avocado, peeled, pitted and cubed
>
> 1 teaspoon garam masala
>
> ½ teaspoon salt
>
> ½ teaspoon cayenne pepper

Directions:

> In a bowl, mix the arugula with the beets and the other ingredients, toss and serve.

Nutrition:

Calories 151

Fat 1.4

Fiber 2.2

Carbs 4.1

Protein 5.9

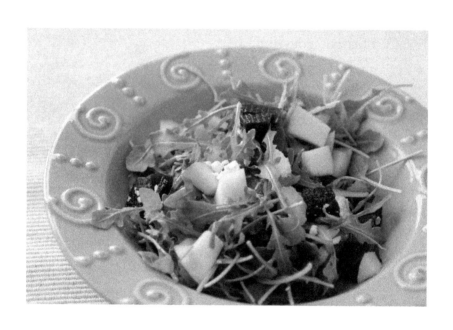

Herbed Beets

Preparation Time: 10 minutes

Cooking Time: 40 minutes

Servings: 3

Ingredients:

- 2 big red beets, peeled and roughly cubed
- 1 tablespoon chives, chopped
- 1 tablespoon cilantro, chopped
- 1 tablespoon basil, chopped
- Juice of 1 lime
- A pinch of salt and black pepper
- ¼ teaspoon dried oregano
- ¼ teaspoon ground nutmeg
- ¼ teaspoon ground cumin
- 1 tablespoon olive oil

Directions:

Spread the beets on a lined baking sheet, add the chives, cilantro and the other ingredients, toss and bake at 400 degrees F for 40 minutes.

Divide between plates and serve.

Nutrition:

Calories 188,Fat 5.2,Fiber 5.9, Carbs 8.3, Protein 1.6

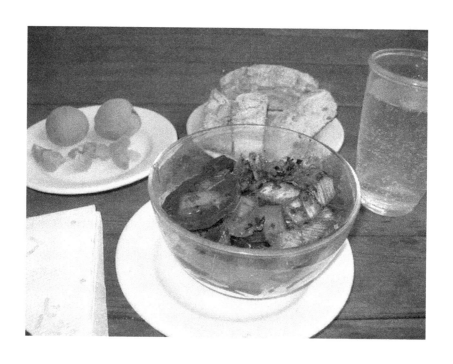

Marinara Broccoli

Preparation Time: 10 minutes

Cooking Time: 15 minutes

Servings: 4

Ingredients:

> 2 cups broccoli florets
>
> 1 teaspoon sweet paprika
>
> 1 teaspoon coriander, ground
>
> ¼ cup marinara sauce
>
> ½ teaspoon ground black pepper
>
> ½ teaspoon salt
>
> ½ teaspoon garlic powder
>
> 1 teaspoon olive oil
>
> Juice of 1 lime

Directions:

> In a roasting pan, mix the broccoli with the marinara
> and the other ingredients, toss and bake at 400
> degrees F for 15 minutes.
>
> Divide between plates and serve.

Nutrition:

Calories206,Fat 4.7,Fiber 3.7,Carbs 10.6, Protein 6.1

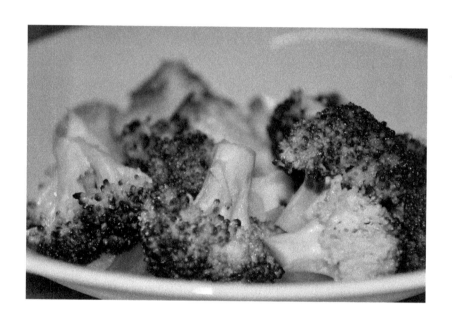

Spinach and Pear Salad

Preparation Time: 10 minutes

Cooking Time: 0 minutes

Servings: 2

Ingredients:

> 1 bell pepper, chopped
>
> ½ cup radishes, halved
>
> ½ cup cherry tomatoes, halved
>
> 2 cups baby spinach
>
> 2 pears, cored and cut into wedges
>
> 1 tablespoon walnuts, chopped
>
> 1 teaspoon chives, chopped
>
> A pinch of salt and black pepper
>
> Juice of 1 lime

Directions:

> In a bowl, mix the radishes with the pepper, tomatoes and the other ingredients, toss and serve.

Nutrition:

Calories 143

Fat 2.9

Fiber 2.1

Carbs 4.9

Protein 3.2

Olives and Mango Mix

Preparation Time: 10 minutes

Cooking Time: 0 minutes

Servings: 2

Ingredients:

> 1 cup black olives, pitted and halved
>
> 1 cup kalamata olives, pitted and halved
>
> 1 cup mango, peeled and cubed
>
> A pinch of salt and black pepper
>
> Juice of 1 lime
>
> 1 teaspoon sweet paprika
>
> 1 teaspoon coriander, ground
>
> 1 tablespoon olive oil

Directions:

> In a bowl mix the olives with the mango and the other ingredients, toss and serve.

Nutrition:

Calories 68

Fat 4.4

Fiber 0

Carbs 1.5

Protein 3.3

Eggplant and Avocado Mix

Preparation Time: 10 minutes
Cooking Time: 20 minutes
Servings: 4

Ingredients:

1 pound eggplant, roughly cubed

2 avocados, peeled, pitted and cubed

1 red onion, chopped

1 teaspoon curry powder

Juice of 1 lime

½ cup crushed tomatoes

1 tablespoon olive oil

1 teaspoon salt

1 teaspoon chili powder

Directions:

Heat up a pan with the oil over medium heat, add the onion and cook for 5 minutes.

Add the eggplants, avocados and the other ingredients, toss and cook for 15 minutes more.

Divide between plates and serve.

Nutrition:

Calories 231,Fat 7.6,Carbs 9.2,Protein 5.4

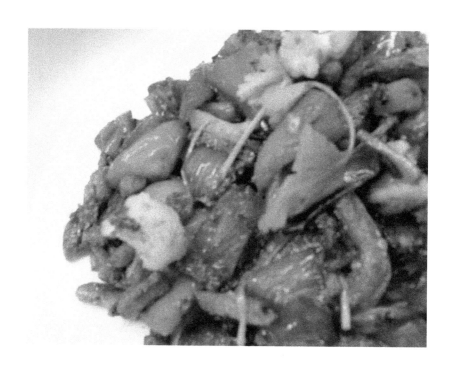

Red Onion, Avocado and Radishes Mix

Preparation Time: 15 minutes

Cooking Time: 12 minutes

Servings: 2

Ingredients:

- 2 red onions, peeled and sliced
- 2 avocados, peeled, pitted and sliced
- 1 cup radishes, halved
- 1 teaspoon oregano, dried
- 1 teaspoon basil, dried
- 1 tablespoon olive oil
- 1 teaspoon lemon juice
- ¼ teaspoon salt

Directions:

Heat up a pan with the oil over medium heat, add the onions, oregano and basil and cook for 5 minutes.
Add the rest of the ingredients, toss, cook for 7 minutes more, divide into bowls and serve.

Nutrition:

Calories 145,Fat 7.1,Fiber 2.4,Carbs 10.3,Protein 6.2

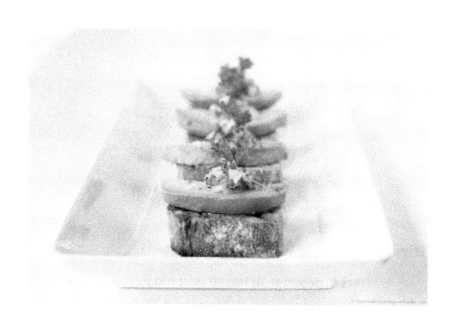

Cajun and Balsamic Okra

Preparation Time: 10 minutes

Cooking Time: 15 minutes

Servings: 2

Ingredients:

1 cup okra, sliced

½ cup crushed tomatoes

1 teaspoon Cajun seasoning

2 tablespoons balsamic vinegar

1 teaspoon salt

1 teaspoon ground black pepper

1 tablespoon fresh parsley, chopped

1 teaspoon olive oil

Directions:

Heat up a pan with the oil over medium heat, add the okra, seasoning and the remaining ingredients, toss and cook for 15 minutes.

Divide into bowls and serve.

Nutrition:

Calories 162

Fat 4.5

Fiber 4.6

Carbs 12.6

Protein 3

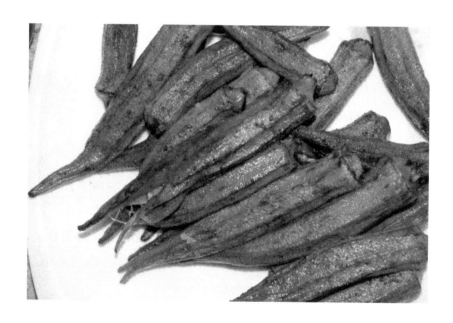

Cashew Zucchinis

Preparation Time: 10 minutes

Cooking Time: 40 minutes

Servings: 4

Ingredients:

> 1 pound zucchinis, sliced
>
> ½ cup cashews, soaked for a couple of hours and drained
>
> 1 cup coconut milk
>
> ¼ teaspoon nutmeg, ground
>
> 1 teaspoon chili powder
>
> A pinch of salt and black pepper

Directions:

In a roasting pan, mix the zucchinis with the cashews and the other ingredients, toss gently and cook at 380 degrees F for 40 minutes.

Divide into bowls and serve.

Nutrition:

Calories 200

Fat 5

Fiber 3

Carbs 7.1

Protein 6.5

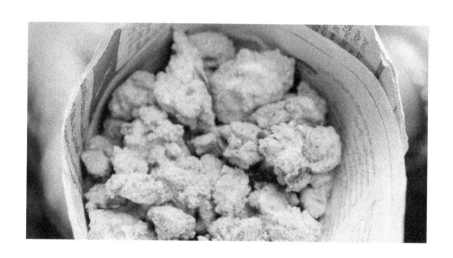

Chili Fennel

Preparation Time: 10 minutes

Cooking Time: 8 minutes

Servings: 4

Ingredients:

- 2 fennel bulbs, cut into quarters
- 3 tablespoons olive oil
- Salt and black pepper to the taste
- 1 garlic clove, minced
- 1 red chili pepper, chopped
- ¾ cup veggie stock
- Juice of ½ lemon

Directions:

1. Heat a pan that fits your Air Fryer with the oil over medium-high heat, add garlic and chili pepper, stir and cook for 2 minutes.
2. Add fennel, salt, pepper, stock, and lemon juice, toss to coat, introduce in your Air Fryer and cook at 350 ° F for at least 6 minutes.
3. Divide into plates and serve as a side dish.

Nutrition:

Calories: 158 kcal ,Protein: 3.57 g ,Fat: 11.94,
Carbohydrates: 11.33 g

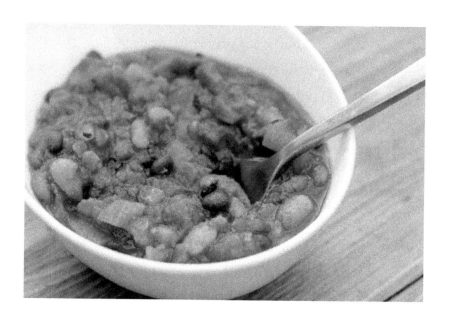

Collard Greens and Tomatoes

Preparation Time: 10 minutes

Cooking Time: 10 minutes

Servings: 9

Ingredients:

- 1 pound collard greens
- ¼ cup cherry tomatoes, halved
- 1 tablespoon apple cider vinegar
- 2 tablespoons veggie stock
- Salt and black pepper to the taste

Directions:

1. In a pan that fits the Air Fryer, combine tomatoes, collard greens, vinegar, stock, salt, and pepper, stir, introduce in your Air Fryer and cook at 320 ° F for 10 minutes.
2. Divide between plates and serve as a side dish.

Nutrition:

Calories: 28 kcal

Protein: 2.34 g

Fat: 0.99 g

Carbohydrates: 3.26 g

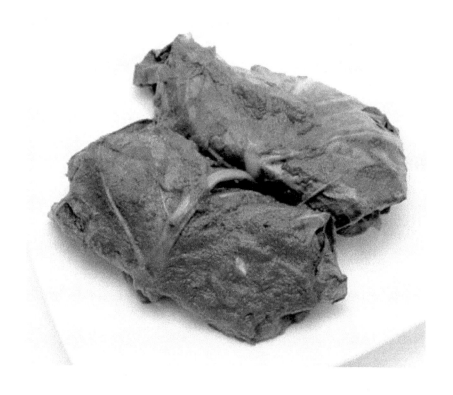

Bean and Carrot Spirals

Preparation Time: 10 minutes

Cooking Time: 40 minutes

Servings: 24

Ingredients:

4 8-inch flour tortillas

1 ½ cups of Easy Mean White Bean dip

10 ounces spinach leaves

½ cup diced carrots

½ cup diced red peppers

Directions:

Starts by preparing the bean dip, seen above. Next, spread out the bean dip on each tortilla, making sure to leave about a ¾ inch white border on the tortillas' surface. Next, place spinach in the center of the tortilla, followed by carrots and red peppers.

Roll the tortillas into tight rolls, and cover every rolls with plastic wrap or aluminum foil.

Let them chill in the fridge for twenty-four hours.

Afterward, remove the wrap from the spirals and remove the very ends of the rolls. Slice the rolls into six individual spiral pieces, and arrange them on a platter for serving. Enjoy!

Nutrition:

Calories: 205 kcal

Protein: 6.41 g

Fat: 4.16 g

Carbohydrates: 35.13 g

Tofu Nuggets with Barbecue Glaze

Preparation Time: 10 minutes

Cooking Time: 25 minutes

Servings: 9

Ingredients:

>32 ounces tofu
>
>1 cup quick vegan barbecue sauce

Directions:

>Set the oven to 425F.
>
>Next, slice the tofu and blot the tofu with clean towels. Next, slice and dice the tofu and completely eliminate the water from the tofu material.
>
>Stir the tofu with the vegan barbecue sauce, and place the tofu on a baking sheet.
>
>Bake the tofu for fifteen minutes. Afterward, stir the tofu and bake the tofu for an additional ten minutes.
>
>Enjoy!

Nutrition:

Calories: 311 kcal

Protein: 19.94 g

Fat: 21.02 g

Carbohydrates: 15.55 g

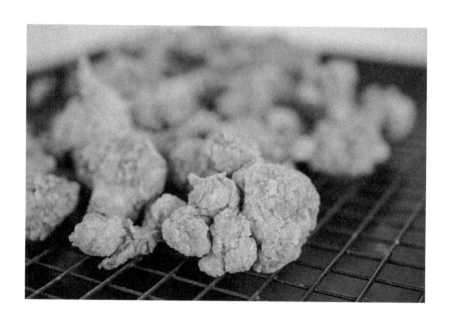

Peppered Pinto Beans

Preparation Time: 10 minutes

Cooking Time: 15 minutes

Servings: 6

Ingredients:

- 1 tsp. Chili powder
- 1 tsp. ground cumin
- .5 cup Vegetable
- 2 cans Pinto beans
- 1 Minced jalapeno
- 1 Diced red bell pepper
- 1 tsp. Olive oil

Directions:

Take out a pot and heat the oil. Cook the jalapeno and pepper for a bit before adding in the pepper, salt, cumin, broth, and beans.

Place to a boil and then reduce the heat to cook for a bit. After 10 minutes, let it cool and serve.

Nutrition:

Calories: 183

Carbs: 32g

Fat: 2g

Protein: 11g

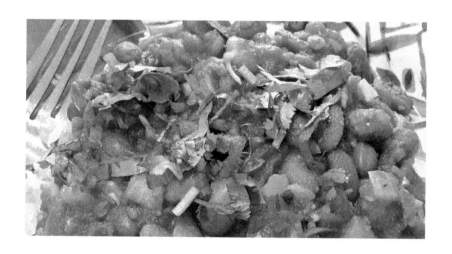

Black Bean Pizza

Preparation Time: 30 minutes

Cooking Time: 20 minutes

Servings: 2

Ingredients:

> 1 Sliced avocado
>
> 1 Sliced red onion
>
> 1 Grated carrot
>
> 1 Sliced tomato
>
> .5 cup Spicy black bean dip
>
> 2 Pizza crusts

Directions:

> Turn on the oven and let heat to 400 degrees. Layout two crusts on a baking sheet and add the dip onto each one.
>
> Top with the tomato slices and sprinkle the carrots and the onion on a well.
>
> Add to the oven and let it bake for about 20 minutes or so until done. Top with the avocado before serving.

Nutrition:

Calories: 379, Carbs: 59g ,Fat: 13g ,Protein: 13g

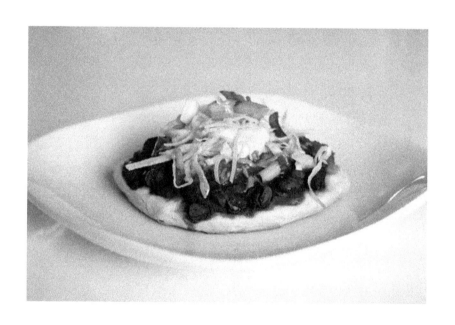

Vegetable and Chickpea Loaf

Preparation Time: 10 minutes

Cooking Time: 15 minutes

Servings: 4

Ingredients:

> 1 tsp. Salt
>
> .5 tsp. Dried sage
>
> 1 tsp. Dried savory
>
> 1 tbsp. Soy sauce
>
> .25 cup Parsley
>
> .5 cup Breadcrumbs
>
> .75 cup Oats
>
> .75 cup Chickpea flour
>
> 1.5 cup cooked chickpeas
>
> 2 Minced garlic cloves
>
> 1 Chopped yellow onion
>
> 1 Shredded carrot
>
> 1 Shredded white potato

Directions:

> Set the oven to 350F. Take out a loaf pan and then grease it up.
>
> Squeeze out the liquid from the potato and add to the food processor with the garlic, onion, and carrot.
>
> Add the chickpeas and pulse to blend well. Add in the rest of the ingredients here, and when it is done,

use your hands to form this into a loaf and add to the pan.

Place into the oven to bake for a bit until it is nice and firm. Let it cool down and then slice.

Nutrition:

Calories: 351 kcal

Protein: 16.86 g

Fat: 6.51 g

Carbohydrates: 64 g

Thyme and Lemon Couscous

Preparation Time: 5 minutes

Cooking Time: 10 minutes

Servings: 6

Ingredients:

.25 cup Chopped parsley

1.5 cup Couscous

2 tbsp. Chopped thyme

Juice and zest of a lemon

2.75 cup Vegetable stock

Directions:

Take out a pot and add in the thyme, lemon juice, and vegetable stock. Stir in the couscous after it has gotten to a boil and then take off the heat.

Allow sitting covered until it can take in all of the liquid. Then fluff up with a form.

Stir in the parsley and lemon zest, then serve warm.

Nutrition:

Calories: 922 kcal

Protein: 2.7 g

Fat: 101.04 g

Carbohydrates: 10.02 g

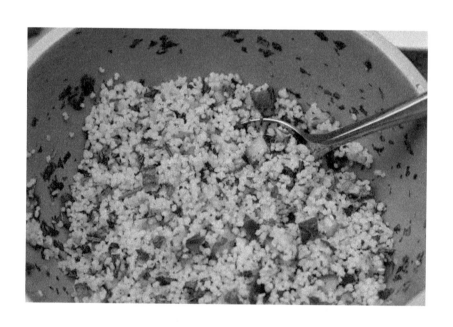

Pesto and White Bean Pasta

Preparation Time: 10 minutes

Cooking Time: 10 minutes

Servings: 4

Ingredients:

> .5 cup Chopped black olives
>
> .25 Diced red onion
>
> 1 cup Chopped tomato
>
> .5 cup Spinach pesto
>
> 1.5 cup Cannellini beans
>
> 8 oz. Rotini pasta, cooked

Directions:

> Bring out a bowl and toss together the pesto, beans, and pasta.
>
> Add in the olives, red onion, and tomato and toss around a bit more before serving.

Nutrition:

Calories 544

Carbs 83g

Fat 17g

Protein 23g

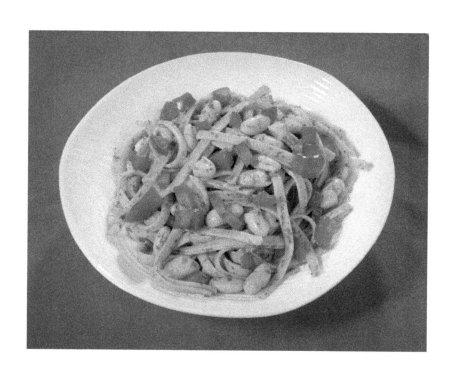

Conclusion

In a nutshell, this cookbook offers you a world full of options to diversify your plant-based menu. People on this diet are usually seen struggling to choose between healthy food and flavor but, soon, they run out of the options. The selection of 250 recipes in this book is enough to adorn your dinner table with flavorsome, plant-based meals every day. Give each recipe a good read and try them out in the kitchen. You will experience tempting aromas and binding flavors every day.

The book is conceptualized with the idea of offering you a comprehensive view of a plant-based diet and how it can benefit the body. You may find the shift sudden, especially if you are a die-hard fan of non-vegetarian items. But you need not give up anything that you love. Eat everything in moderation.

The next step is to start experimenting with the different recipes in this book and see which ones are your favorites. Everyone has their favorite food, and you will surely find several of yours in this book. Start with breakfast and work your way through. You will be pleasantly surprised at how tasty a vegan meal really can be.

You will love reading this book, as it helps you to understand how revolutionary a plant-based diet can be. It will help you to make informed decisions as you move toward greater change for the greater good. What are you waiting for? Have you begun your journey on the path of the plant-based diet yet? If you haven't, do it now!

Now you have everything you need to get started making budget-friendly, healthy plant-based recipes. Just follow your basic shopping list and follow your meal plan to get started! It's easy to switch over to a plant-based diet if you have your meals planned out and temptation locked away. Don't forget to clean out your kitchen before starting, and you're sure to meet all your diet and health goals.

You need to plan if you are thinking about dieting. First, you can start slowly by just eating one meal a day, which is vegetarian and gradually increasing your number of vegetarian meals. Whenever you are struggling, ask your friend or family member to support you and keep you motivated. One important thing is also to be regularly accountable for not following the diet.

If dieting seems very important to you and you need to do it right, then it is recommended that you visit a professional such as a nutritionist or dietitian to discuss your dieting plan and optimizing it for the better.

No matter how much you want to lose weight, it is not advised that you decrease your calorie intake to an unhealthy level. Losing weight does not mean that you stop eating. It is done by carefully planning meals.

A plant-based diet is very easy once you get into it. At first, you will start to face a lot of difficulties, but if you start slowly, then you can face all the barriers and achieve your goal.

Swap out one unhealthy food item each week that you know is not helping you and put in its place one of the plant-based ingredients that you like. Then have some fun creating the many different recipes in this book. Find out what recipes you like the most so you can make them often and most of all; have some fun exploring all your recipe options.

Wish you good luck with the plant-based diet!

CPSIA information can be obtained
at www.ICGtesting.com
Printed in the USA
BVHW041741120421
604749BV00014B/430